WS

310

SCH

NLM

D1357212

Springer

Berlin
Heidelberg
New York
Hong Kong
London
Milan
Paris
Tokyo

Felix Schier

Laparoscopy in Children

With Contributions by
Keith Georgeson (Birmingham/Alabama, USA)
and David van der Zee (Utrecht, Netherlands)

With 67 Figures in 165 Separate Illustrations

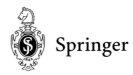

Professor Dr. Felix Schier
Abteilung für Kinderchirurgie
Friedrich-Schiller-Universität
Bachstrasse 18, 07743 Jena, Germany
email: felix.schier@med.uni-jena.de

ISBN 3-540-42975-1 Springer-Verlag Berlin Heidelberg New York

Library of Congress Cataloging-in-Publication Data
Schier, F. Laparoscopy in children/Schier, Felix; with contributions by Keith Georgeson and David van der Zee. p.; cm. Includes index.
ISBN 3540429751 (hardcover: alk. paper)
1. Children-Surgery. 2. Laparoscopic surgery. I. Title.
[DNLM: 1. Laparoscopy-methods-Child. 2. Abdomen-surgery-Child. WS 310 S332L 2003]
RD137.S285 2003 617.5'5059'083-dc21 2002030218

This work is subject to copyright. All rights are reserved, whether the whole or part of the material is concerned, specifically the rights of translation, reprinting, reuse of illustrations, recitation, broadcasting, reproduction on microfilm or in any other way, and storage in data banks. Duplication of this publication or parts thereof is permitted only under the provision of the German Copyright Law of September 9, 1965, in its current version, and permission for use must always be obtained from Springer-Verlag. Violations are liable for prosecution under the German Copyright Law.

Springer-Verlag Berlin Heidelberg New York
a member of BertelsmannSpringer Science + Business Media GmbH
http://www.springer.de

© Springer-Verlag Berlin Heidelberg 2003
Printed in Germany

The use of designations, trademarks, etc. in this publication does not imply, even in the absence of a specific statement, that such names are exempt from the relevant protective laws and regulations and therefore free for general use.

Product liability: The publisher cannot guarantee the accuracy of any information about dosage and application contained in this book. In every individual case the user must check such information by consulting the relevant literature.

Cover-Design: Erich Kirchner, Springer-Verlag, Heidelberg
Typesetting: Data conversion by Springer-Verlag Heidelberg
Printing: Saladruck GmbH, Berlin
Bookbinding: Stürtz AG, Würzburg
Printed on acid-free paper.   SPIN 10843353   24/3150 ih - 5 4 3 2 1 0

Contents

Introduction

Laparoscopy in children is a special technique. Children come in all sizes, and the fact that children are small is an important technical aspect. In addition, there are characteristic pediatric indications for laparoscopy. The most typical ones are described here.

This booklet was written for colleagues - adult and pediatric surgeons alike - wishing to profit from the experience of authors who have performed numerous laparoscopies in children of all sizes, many of them newborns.

The authors are aware of the fact that current medical progress may appear ridiculous in 100 years. Laparoscopy in children only began 10 years ago, and techniques are constantly changing. Readers should thus see our comments as preliminary ones. Any suggestions for improvements would be very welcome.

All humans have a healthy natural inhibition about inserting sharp instruments into a small child's abdomen. However, once they have cut through the abdominal wall and can find their bearings, surgeons usually feel comfortable.

Two problems remain, namely bleeding control and suturing. These are particular problems in laparoscopy. In children, however, there are almost no interventions with a serious risk of bleeding (except splenectomy). Suturing is seldom required in children (except in fundoplication and inguinal hernia).

This booklet contains no statistics and no comparisons with open approaches. Instead, it concentrates on the practical steps involved. Applying the techniques described, the reader may also master procedures not mentioned here. The principles are covered in this booklet.

Do not use 10-mm instruments in children. Complete sets of instruments of 2 or 3 mm in diameter or even less are available. They enable us to operate virtually without scars and can also be used in adults.

Take children seriously. Surgeons need practice, and so does the rest of the team.

Good luck!   Felix Schier
                              e-mail: felix.schier@med.uni-jena.de

The Trolley

2 Standard equipment is used: monitor, video equipment, insufflator, light source etc.
Two pieces of equipment need special attention:

- The insufflator has to be capable of delivering volumes of CO_2 of less than 0.5 l/min. Many insufflators will only work at rates of 1 l/min or more. A small child may only have a capacity of 150 ml. Insufflation is completed in seconds. CO_2 does not need to be heated. Temperature loss is only a concern if trocars fall out and instruments are changed excessively often. (This requires re-insufflation with cool CO_2).
- The light source needs to be powerful. As much light as possible has to be squeezed through narrow trocars.

All the remaining equipment is standard, as used in adult laparoscopy. The cautery is the piece of equipment that most often fails.
The trolley should be placed on the other side of the patient, with the patient between the surgeon and the trolley.
In contrast to conventional arrangements, place the monitor low in order to close the angle between working and looking directions.

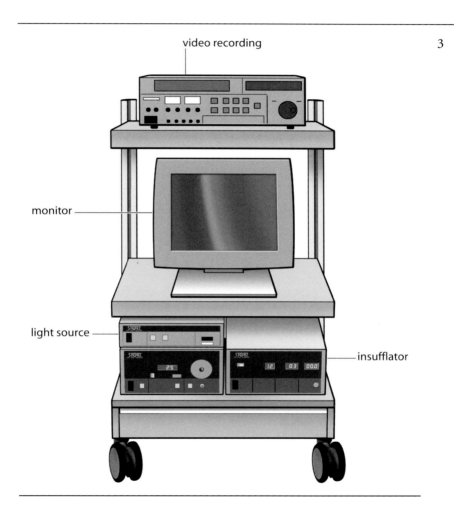

The Patient

4   A urinary catheter is unnecessary, as a full bladder seldom obstructs the view. If it does, a large-bore needle can be inserted through the abdominal wall to empty the bladder. Children should go to the toilet before laparoscopy.

Enemas are unnecessary. They will not necessarily empty the colon and may even distend it.

Padding below the patient is risky, as it lifts up the endangered vessels and brings the structures upward into the reach of the trocars.

Laparoscopy is easier if the patient is fully relaxed.

The small and large bowels are often dilated in small children, making visualization difficult.

The child should be prepared such that conversion to an open approach is possible at any time.

Put a neutral electrode in place in order to save time if conversion becomes necessary.

Adjust the ether screen to a low position in order to reach the pelvis with the laparoscope.

Prior to introducing the first trocar, prepare the laparoscope in order to be able to see immediately after the trocar is inserted; furthermore, check that the cautery is functioning properly with a wet sponge prior to inserting the first trocar.

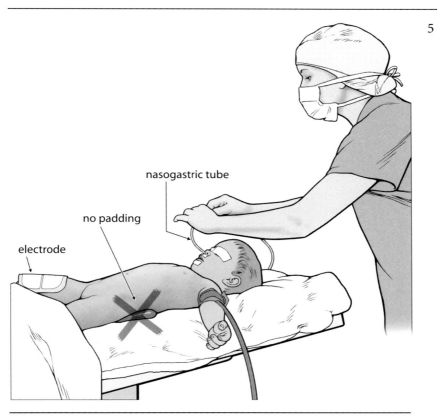

6   Laparoscopy

Premedicate the patient with a parasympatholytic (this reduces the likelihood of bradycardia and bronchial hypersecretion).

For monitoring, use capnography, pulse oximetry, non-invasive blood pressure measuring and electrocardiography (ECG).

Insert a nasogastric tube (this prevents trocar perforation and aspiration).

Use volatile anesthetics, and remember the association between halothane and arrhythmias in hypercapnia. Isoflurane or sevoflurane should be preferred (less myocardial depression). Avoid nitrous oxide (thought to distend the bowel).

Use tracheal intubation and controlled ventilation. Check the position of the tracheal tube again after CO_2 insufflation (when the diaphragm is elevated, there is a relative downshift of the tube, producing a risk of unilateral intubation).

Adjust ventilation to end-tidal CO_2, increase ventilation up to 60% (mainly via the respiratory rate), and maintain a positive end-expiratory pressure (PEEP) of 3-5 cm H_2O (this prevents microatelectases and intrapulmonary shunting).

Continued on p. 8

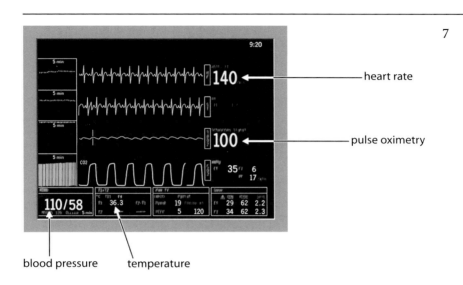

heart rate

pulse oximetry

blood pressure   temperature

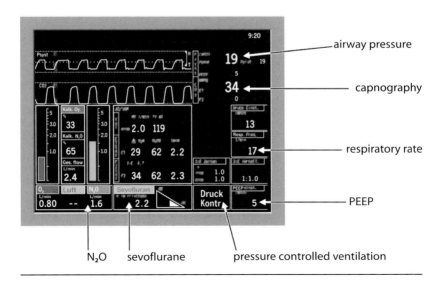

airway pressure

capnography

respiratory rate

PEEP

N₂O   sevoflurane   pressure controlled ventilation

8   Thoracoscopy

Controlled ventilation with single-lung ventilation:
- Neonates: intubate into one main bronchus.
- Infants: combine conventional endotracheal tubes with a "bronchial blocker".
- Children heavier than 20 kg: use special tubes with an integrated bronchial blocker (Univent-Tube, Fuji Systems, Japan).
- Children heavier than 30 kg: use regular double-lumen tracheal tubes (Broncho-Cath, Mallinckrodt, Ireland).

Fiberoptic bronchoscopy is required (check the tube position, and evacuate pus and blood).

Continued on p. 10

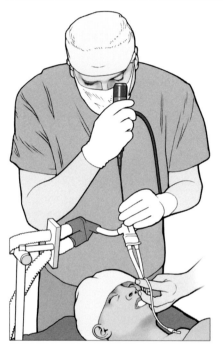

bronchoscopy

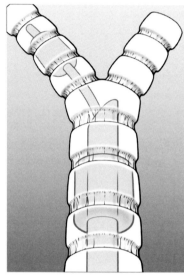

single lung ventilation

10   Gas Embolism

CO_2 enters the venous system and the right ventricle, blocking the pulmonary vasculature. This leads to right heart failure, dilated neck veins, hypotension, bradycardia, desaturation, CO_2 retention (but low end-tidal CO_2 pressure, $PEtCO_2$) and a rise in airway pressure. This has never been seen by the author.

Action to be taken
1. Stop CO_2 insufflation.
2. Stop nitrous oxide (this reduces bubble size), and administer 100% O2.
3. Perform Durant's maneuver: left-sided head-down position (this shifts pulmonary outflow, with gas bubbles accumulating above, and restores adequate cardiac output).

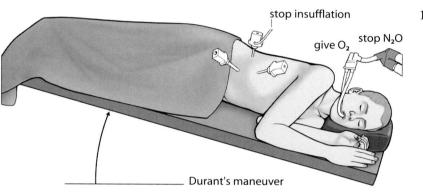

Insufflation (1)

12   Make a 4-mm transverse incision below the lower rim of the umbilicus so that the incision is later hidden inside the umbilicus. This also saves a skin suture later when withdrawing the trocar.

Spread the tissue with small scissors down to the fascia.

Insert a Veres needle while lifting up the abdominal wall on both sides. There are two distinct snaps – both of them visible, audible, and palpable – when inserting the Veres needle. The second structure, the peritoneum, is the more resistant one.

Stay inside the umbilicus, because there are fewer structures to be crossed here. Do not aim toward the bladder.

Estimate how deep you are by tilting the needle and palpating for the tip.

Insufflation (1)

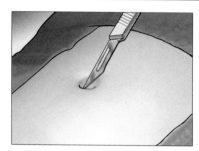

incision

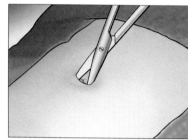

spread with scissors

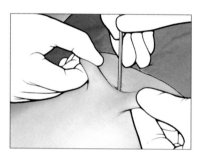

lift abdominal wall for insertion of
Veres needle

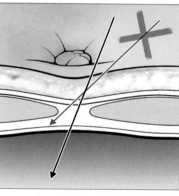

stay within anatomy of umbilicus

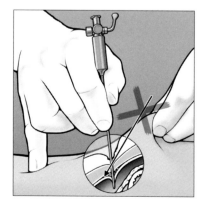

palpate needle end

14   First inject physiologic saline in order to rule out high resistance as in intramuscular injection. Aspirate to rule out intravascular placement.

Perform the "hanging drop test": fill the Veres needle with physiologic saline and lift up the abdominal wall: saline is sucked into the abdomen. This is considered proof that the needle tip is located intraperitoneally.

The following insufflation rates should be used:
-   <1 year: 0.3 l/min
-   >1 year: 0.5 l/min
-   >5 years: 1 l/min
-   >10 years: 2 l/min

Start with 0.5 l/min until you are sure that the needle has been inserted intraperitoneally.

Pressure will initially be -2 to +3 mmHg and will slowly increase. Continue pulling up the abdominal wall (this prevents occlusion of the needle tip with the omentum). Initial pressures of 13-17 mmHg indicate that the needle is in the wrong position (most likely outside the peritoneum); it should be withdrawn and reinserted. The maximum pressure is 12 mmHg for all age-groups. In children older than 10 years, 15 mmHg is acceptable, but this may result in postoperative shoulder pain. Visualization will not be reduced when the pressure is lowered to 8 mmHg.

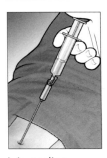

inject saline,
aspirate

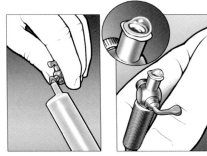

"hanging drop test": 1. fill needle
with saline

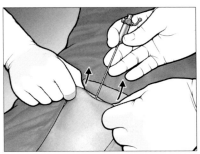

2. lift abdominal wall

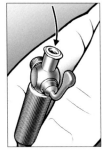

3. drop will be
sucked in

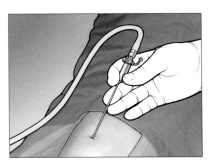

insufflate

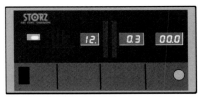

pressure initially -2 to +3
max. pressure: 12, flow: 0.3

Trocar Insertion

16   A 5-mm trocar is inserted at the umbilicus for the laparoscope. Be sure to have the valves closed and the safety mechanism activated (if the valves are open, the CO_2 will escape immediately upon entering the abdominal cavity). Guard the forearm to prevent rushing in too deeply. When inserting the trocar, lift up the abdominal wall bilaterally.

Insert the laparoscope and check its position. If it is correct, begin insufflation.

Continued on p. 18

Trocar Insertion

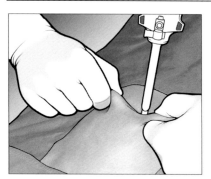

insert trocar

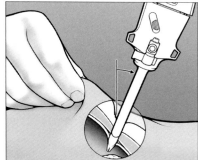

sligthly oblique

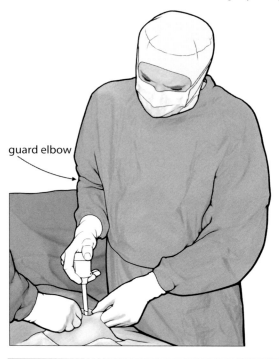

guard elbow

Trocar Insertion

18   Place the next trocars away from the target organ, not directly on top of it. The line between the target organ, the trocar, and the instrument should be considered as an extension of the surgeon's forearm.

Once the laparoscope has been inserted into the abdominal cavity, remember that the space is small, the bowel is dilated (especially in small children), and the view is close. All these factors make the initial orientation difficult.

The laparoscope is usually inserted through the umbilicus, except in fundoplication and sigmoid resection. In fundoplication, the view is better if the laparoscope is inserted higher up, half-way between the umbilicus and the xiphoid process. In sigmoid resection, the view is better if the laparoscope is inserted away from the center, in the right upper abdomen.

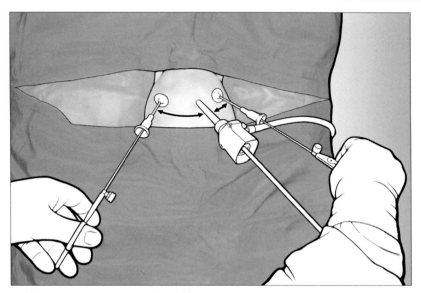

working trocars apart, extension of forearm

Instruments

20   We use 5-mm/0° laparoscopes, 30° laparoscopes are more difficult
to handle. Fogging can be prevented by increasing the light inten-
sity to 100% before inserting the laparoscope. This heats the tip of
the laparoscope. Alternatively, anti-fogging solution can be used.
Keep the laparoscope as far away as possible from the target organ.
This facilitates orientation.
Five-millimeter instruments and trocars are too large to be used in
small children. Sets of 3-mm, 2-mm, and even 1-mm instruments
are available; 2-mm instruments are easily bent and broken, but
3-mm instruments are sturdy.

Continued on p. 21

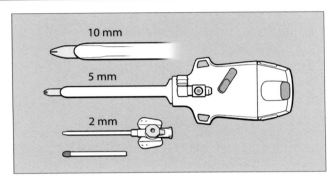

trocars

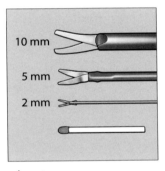

scissors

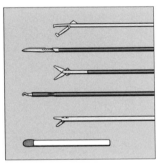

various 2-mm instruments

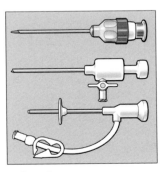

various 2-mm trocars

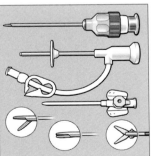

instruments for herniotomy

Instruments

22   Trocars for 3-mm instruments are still rather large. Trocars for 2-mm instruments are significantly smaller, and they do not need any suturing upon withdrawal; a bandage suffices. Instruments with a diameter of 1.7 mm fit no. 12 hypodermic needles and therefore do even not require a formal trocar. However, they tend to fall out if the instrument is removed too quickly. In addition, when the jaws of the instruments are opened, even only slightly, the trocars will fall out.

Suction and irrigation is useful with 5-mm laparoscopes. Suction is unnecessary with 2-mm instruments, as the fluid will be expressed through the cannula due to the increased intraabdominal pressure.

The cosmetic results achieved with 2-mm instruments are superb, and there are virtually no scars. Two-millimeter clips are not available, and tied ligatures have to be used with 2-mm instruments.

The 5-mm entry port at the umbilicus is closed with an absorbable 4-0 fascia suture.

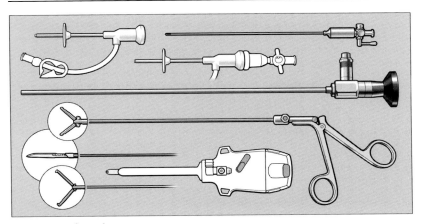

instruments for pyloromyotomy

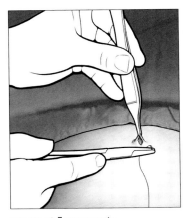

suture at 5-mm ports

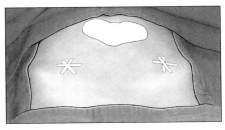

Steristrips at 2-mm ports

Ligating

24   Pre-tied endoloops should be used. Pass the endoloop through the trocar using an introducer (otherwise the loop bends and is difficult to insert). Commercial introducers are available, but you can make your own by using the guider from commercially available endoloops and making the knot yourself. This reduces costs. The principle of the knot is easy to remember.

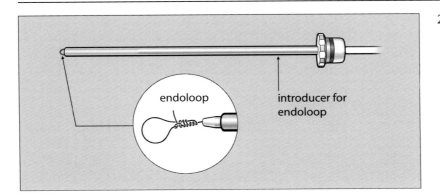

endoloop

introducer for
endoloop

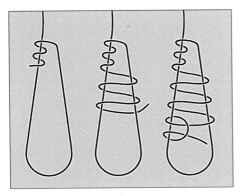

principle of endoloop knot

Needle Insertion

---

26 Insert the needle though 5-mm trocars or, if you are using 2-mm trocars, directly through the abdominal wall. Finish suturing and eventually remove the sutures together with a trocar. Needles for 5-0 or 6-0 sutures may be removed through 2-mm trocars.

Needle Insertion

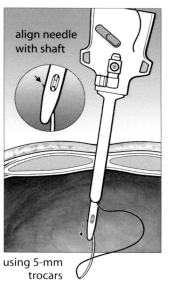

align needle with shaft

using 5-mm trocars

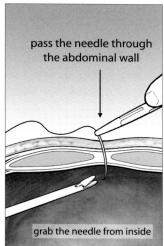

pass the needle through the abdominal wall

grab the needle from inside

using 2-mm trocars

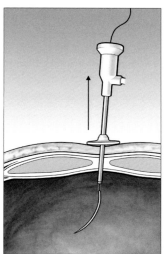

removal of the needle (together with trocar

Suturing

28   Suturing is initially tedious and frustrating, but practice helps. Use intracorporeal knotting, which is easier because it is similar to "open" instrument knotting.

Use two needle holders, especially when using 2-mm needle holders. The left hand has a firmer grip with a needle holder. Use a ratched needle holder for your right hand and a non-ratched needle holder for your left (or the other way round if you are left-handed). Use regular sutures as for open surgery. 4-0 sutures and needle sizes of 18-20 mm are adequate for small children. Using 2-mm needle holders, even 7-0 sutures may be used without difficulty. To make the suture pass through a 5-mm trocar, bend open the needle a little. Cut the length of the suture to approximately 7 cm, depending on the size of the abdominal cavity (the smaller the cavity, the shorter the suture), and make the stitch. Keep the needle in your right hand so that the needle end points toward you and the thread end points away. Look for the free end of the suture. Rotate the thread end of the needle with your right hand around the (open) jaws in your left - just as you would in open instrument knotting. Leave a short free end. Hold the needle in your left hand; hold it at the tip and have the tip point away from you and the thread end toward you. Again, the (open) jaws in your right hand are rotated around the thread end.

Remember that sutures are easily ruptured inside (law of levers).

intracorporeal suturing

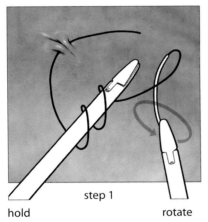 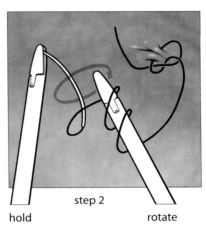

step 1

step 2

hold   rotate   hold   rotate

Adhesiolysis

30   Place the child in a high position because surgery will be performed "at the ceiling".
Forceps are required to stretch the bands, bipolar forceps for coagulation, and scissors to transect the coagulated adhesion.

Continued on p. 32

Adhesiolysis

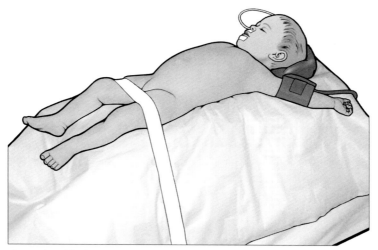

elevated positioning

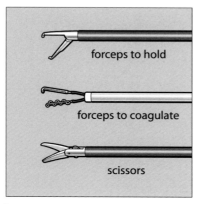

forceps to hold

forceps to coagulate

scissors

instruments

Adhesiolysis

32 Keep the first trocar away from the scar. In adhesions, we prefer the "open" Hasson technique to ensure that we do not perforate adherent bowel. (Otherwise we use the Veres needle approach). Most experienced laparoscopists have perforated adherent bowel at some stage of their career, including the author.

Keep the laparoscope as far away as possible from anticipated adhesions. The extent and density of adhesions are difficult to evaluate if they are immediately in front of the optic.

The size of the scar does not give any indication of the extent of adhesions. Some adhesions are very limited and easy to transect, while others are widespread and densely adherent. If a straightforward transection is not feasible, we do not hesitate to convert and reopen the old scar. There is no point in insisting on a minimally invasive technique if there is already a scar.

Continued on p. 34

Adhesiolysis

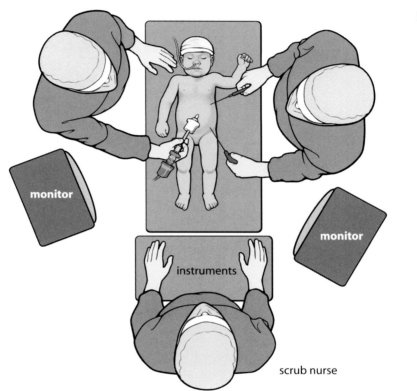

theater layout - trocar placement

Adhesiolysis

34 We coagulate the bands before performing transection. The majority of the bands contain blood vessels. Beginners risk incising too close to the abdominal wall, thereby removing the peritoneum over extended areas.

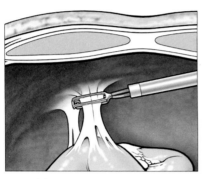

coagulate

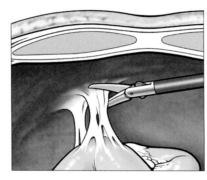

cut

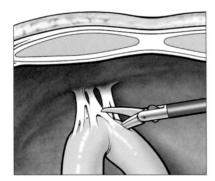

beware of bowel perforation

Appendectomy

36   We use two different techniques, the classical three-trocar technique and the single-trocar technique. The single-trocar technique is preferable for uncomplicated appendectomies. Either technique may be performed with one or two monitors.

The instruments used are forceps with teeth (and a ratched handle) to hold the tip of the appendix, bipolar coagulation forceps to coagulate the mesoappendix, scissors to transect the coagulated mesoappendix and the appendix, and two or three endoloops to ligate the base of the appendix.

Continued on p. 38

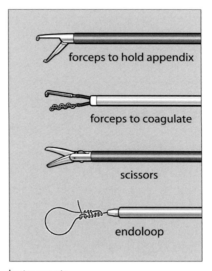

forceps to hold appendix

forceps to coagulate

scissors

endoloop

instruments

Appendectomy

38 **Three Trocar Technique**

A 5-mm/0° laparoscope is inserted at the umbilicus. Two further trocars are inserted in the right and left lower or middle lower abdomen. The left trocar is either 2 or 5 mm in diameter, and the right trocar is 5 mm for a 5-year-old child and 10 mm for a 10-year-old child.

Continued on p. 40

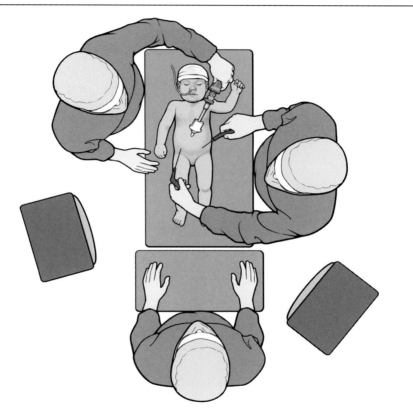

theater layout - trocar placement / "classical", two monitors

Appendectomy

40   In both techniques, the tip of the appendix is grabbed and is pulled
      into and rotated within the right trocar in such a way that the
      mesoappendix is facing the surgeon. The mesocolon is coagulated
      directly towards the base in several steps. Each step is followed by
      cutting with scissors. Coagulate more than you cut, and do not cut
      into non-coagulated tissue.

Continued on p. 42

Appendectomy

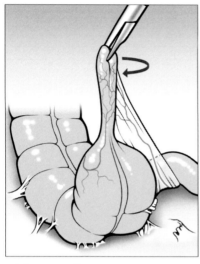

rotate appendix

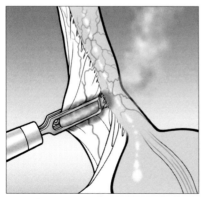

coagulate

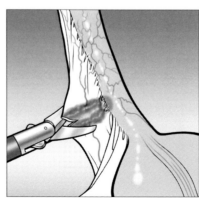

cut meso

Appendectomy

42   The skeletized appendix is ligated with three polydioxanone (PDS) endoloops. The first is placed near the base, and the appendix is then coagulated distally at the level of subsequent transection. An additional endoloop is placed at the base, and a third one more distally. The appendix is cut in between and removed through the trocar. The stump is coated with Betadine solution.

Continued on p. 44

Appendectomy

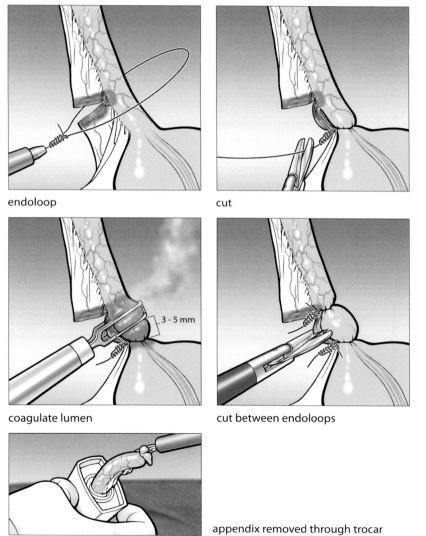

endoloop

cut

coagulate lumen

3 - 5 mm

cut between endoloops

appendix removed through trocar

Appendectomy

---

44   Single-Trocar Technique

A 10-mm trocar is inserted at the umbilicus. The angulated laparoscope with an in-built 5-mm working channel is inserted. Long
and short versions are available, but only the short version can be
used for regular 5-mm instruments. The long version of a co-axial
laparoscope requires "extra-long" 5-mm instruments. In addition,
the endoloops can only be used in the short version.

Continued on p. 46

Appendectomy

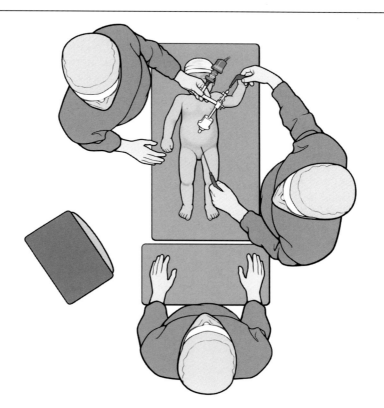

theater layout - trocar placement / "single trocar", one monitor

Appendectomy

46 To manipulate and expose the appendix, use an additional (or two additional) 1.7- or 2-mm instruments inserted in the suprapubic area likely to be covered later by pubic hair. This helps to hold the appendix and place the endoloops. The remaining steps are identical to the classical technique. Remove the appendix using the 10-mm trocar.

Retrocecal appendices are more easily removed laparoscopically. This takes time, however. We would advise against laparoscopic techniques in obvious appendiceal "masses." "Open" abscess drainage appears more logical, and the surgeon's finger preserves more tissue in these cases.

In perforated appendicitis, thorough irrigation is easier to achieve laparoscopically. We use several liters for irrigation. Fecoliths are easily lost and difficult to find in laparoscopy; they also break easily.

"single trocar"

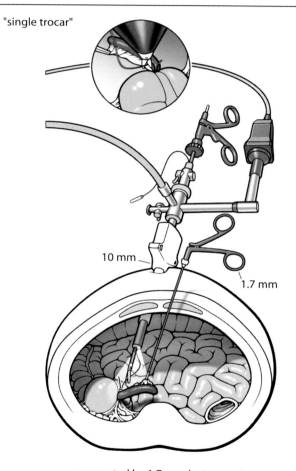

10 mm

1.7 mm

supported by 1.7-mm instrument

Cholecystectomy (With or Without Clips)

48   The laparoscope is inserted through the umbilicus. The surgeon stands either between the patient's legs or on the left side. The procedure is quicker using 5-mm instruments, and clips may be used with this size of instrument. We dislike the use of clips in children in principle and ligate the vessels with 4-0 absorbable ligatures. We prefer using 2-mm instruments for cosmetic reasons.

Continued on p. 50

Cholecystectomy (With or Without Clips)

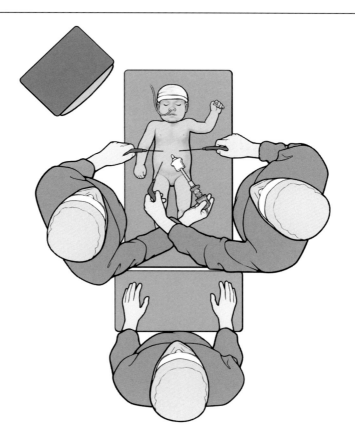

theater layout - trocar placement

Cholecystectomy (With or Without Clips)

50 The instruments required are forceps (with a ratched handle) to push up the gallbladder, forceps to stretch the serosa above the vessels, scissors for coagulation, and two needle holders for ligating the vessels. A 2-mm hook (analogous to the 5-mm hook) is available. It is quicker to perform coagulation and transection using scissors, although they tend to become blunt with this technique.

The fundus of the gallbladder is grasped and pushed cranially. The neck of the bladder is pulled to the right.

Continued on p. 52

Cholecystectomy (With or Without Clips)

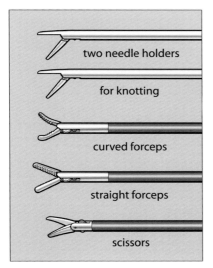

two needle holders

for knotting

curved forceps

straight forceps

scissors

instruments

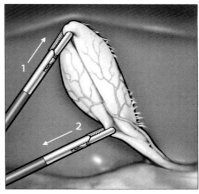

1. push up bladder, 2. expose triangle

Cholecystectomy (With or Without Clips)

52 The peritoneum is opened longitudinally and the vessels are exposed, ligated, and transected.
The gallbladder is gradually freed from its bed by pulling and transecting the remaining ligaments. Finally, the gallbladder is aspirated to reduce the volume and removed through the umbilicus.

Cholecystectomy (With or Without Clips)

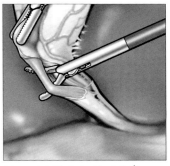

open serosa, expose vessels

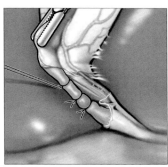

ligate duct

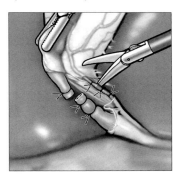

idem with artery

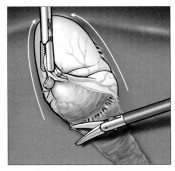

incise laterally

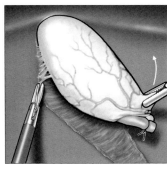

twist bladder to expose lateral attachments

Cholecystectomy

54 We have opened the gallbladder, removed a single stone, and closed the bladder with a running suture in several children. This appears justified in children without a history of metabolic disturbances or a risk of formation of new stones.

"Fishing" with forceps in the opened gallbladder leads to gall spillage. We lost the stone in the bladder twice when trying to extract it. We suggest placing a small sponge (inserted through the 5-mm trocar at the umbilicus) below the bladder opening, preventing the stone from falling between the bowel loops.

Cholecystectomy

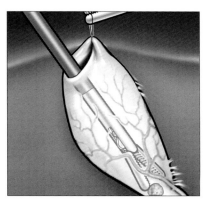

extract the stone ...

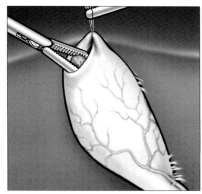

... with forceps

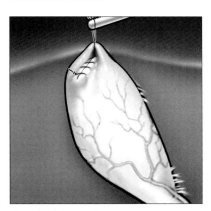

closed with running suture

Cryptorchidism

Statistically, surgeons will encounter the following situations. These are only approximate figures, given in order to prepare surgeons for what they should expect.

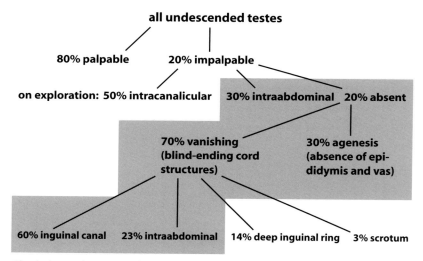

Shaded area: laparoscopic approach indicated

The laparoscope is inserted at the umbilicus. The monitor is placed at the affected side, opposite the surgeon.

Continued on p. 58

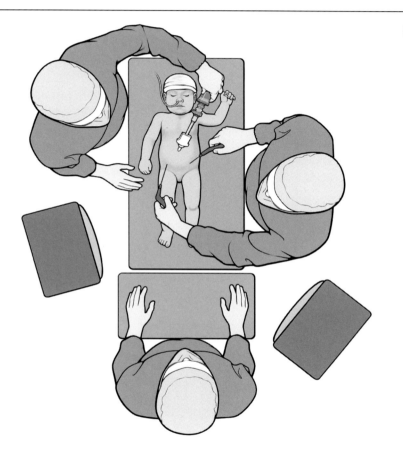

theater layout - trocar placement

Cryptorchidism

58   The instruments required are blunt forceps to hold the testicle, scissors to open the serosa (if required), and two needle holders in case the vessels need to be ligated. All instruments are 2 mm in diameter.

The inner inguinal ring is usually open, and the testis is readily found somewhere nearby or in the canal. If in doubt, a small trocar can be inserted at the lateral abdominal wall, ipsilateral to the affected side (in left-sided cryptorchidism, the trocar is inserted in the left abdomen, for example). The testis will be found just inside the inguinal canal.

A closed process often indicates absent or vanishing testis.

In that case, an additional further trocar should be inserted in order to have one trocar for each hand. In right-sided cryptorchidism, one trocar should be inserted just above the bladder and another lateral to the right rectus sheath, for example. Grab the peritoneum and make a small incision above the vessels.

Continued on p. 60

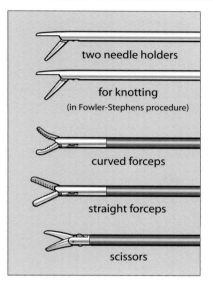

two needle holders

for knotting
(in Fowler-Stephens procedure)

curved forceps

straight forceps

scissors

instruments

findings

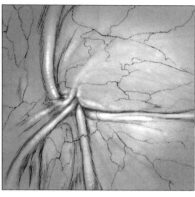

ring closed (= no testis)

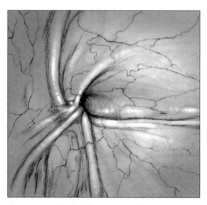

ring open (= testis present)

Cryptorchidism

60   Follow the vessels (blood vessels and vas) to the distal blind ending. There is either a nubbing or a fibrous strand. Resect the nubbing and obtain histology.
If unable to follow the vessels to the very end, convert to an open inguinal exploration.

Continued on p. 62

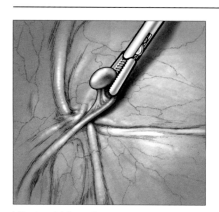

blind nubbing of vas

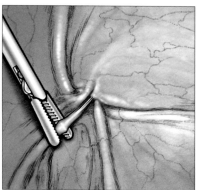

fibrotic end of vas

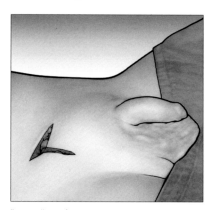

"open" exploration

Cryptorchidism

62   In the case of a low intraabdominal testis, check laparoscopically as to whether the testis is mobile: if it can be mobilized to the contralateral inner ring using forceps, it can be transferred down into the scrotum without any difficulty. Use a conventional, open orchiopexy for this second step.

In high intraabdominal testis before puberty and in patients with bilateral high intraabdominal testis, laparoscopic ligation of the testicular vessels should be performed. This is followed 4-6 months later by laparoscopic transection and conventional orchiopexy (staged Fowler-Stephens procedure). The ligature should remain cranial to the testis. If transected immediately, the testis will spontaneously descend to the internal ring, where it can be brought down through a conventional groin incision now or later (without a second laparoscopy). We dislike using clips and prefer to ligate with absorbable suture material.

In high intraabdominal testis after puberty with normal contralateral scrotal testis or with poor testicular quality, laparoscopic orchiectomy should be performed. If there is only one testis, microvascular transfer should be carried out.

Continued on p. 64

Cryptorchidism

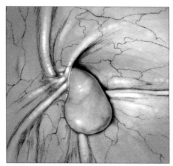

low intraabdominal

Fowler-Stephens

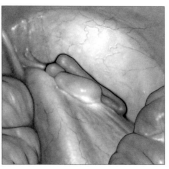

high intraabdominal

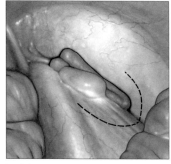

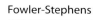

incision

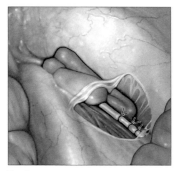

ligatures

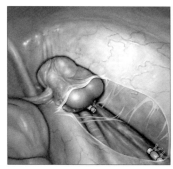

transection

Cryptorchidism

64   To diagnose "vanishing testis" or "agenesis," compare the vessels with the contralateral side. No further exploration is required, and the procedure is complete.

vanishing testis

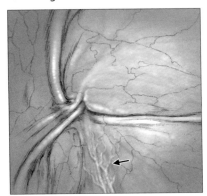 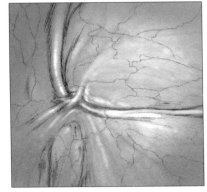

fading vessels   absence of vas and epididymis

Fundoplication (360° Nissen)

66   Pass the laparoscope superior to the umbilicus (closer to the xiphoid process). A 30° laparoscope may be better than 0°. Position the trocar for the liver retractor to the right of the xiphoid process, and place additional trocars in the left and right abdomen. The surgeon may stand at the right, at the left, or between the patient's legs, although we prefer to stand at the right. Place the monitor opposite the surgeon.

Continued on p. 68

Fundoplication (360° Nissen)

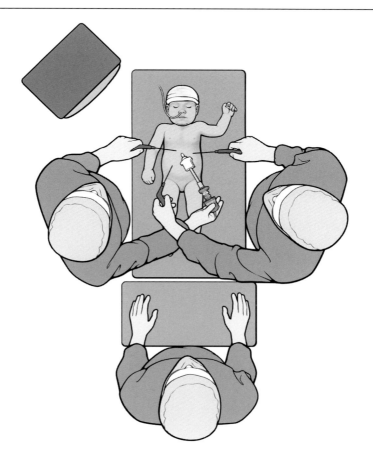

theater layout - trocar placement

Fundoplication (360° Nissen)

68 We use a three-digit 5-mm liver retractor (Lawton). Retractors are available which can be bent inside. The abdomen is pulled down through an additional trocar in the left middle/lower abdomen. Coagulation forceps are used to transect the connective tissue right through to the stomach. Two needle holders are better for suturing than one needle holder and forceps. In principle, we prefer 2-mm instruments for all procedures. Fundoplication, however, is better performed using 5-mm instruments, as they are mechanically more sturdy.

The transverse colon is dilated in many children. You should continue the procedure, as it will collapse later.

Obtain an overview of the patient's anatomy: expose the hiatus and the right limb of the diaphragmatic crus.

Apply downward traction on the stomach. Stretch and coagulate the phrenoesophageal ligament. Leave the opening small because it may contain the left hepatic artery or hepatic branches of the vagus nerve and can subsequently be used to stabilize the wrap.

Directly below the opening is the right limb of the crus. Peel off the fascial layer of the crus (it does not need to be cut in small children). Do not fully expose the muscle fibres since sutures may cut through.

Enter the space between the crus and esophagus by blunt dissection. Position a sling, as in open surgery.

Continued on p. 70

Fundoplication (360° Nissen)

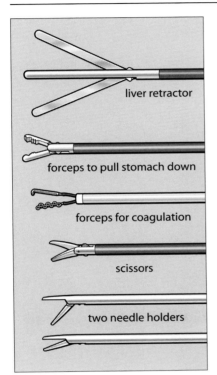

liver retractor

forceps to pull stomach down

forceps for coagulation

scissors

two needle holders

instruments

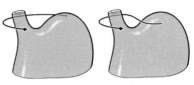

Nissen   Rosetti

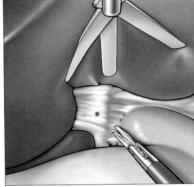

identify right crus

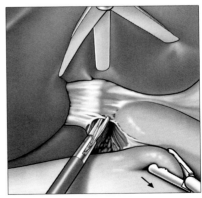

pull down stomach, open ligament

Fundoplication (360° Nissen)

70   Pull the esophagus to the right. Expose the left limb of the crus, again by blunt peeling. Expose the esophagus proximally (for a few centimeters), and pull the esophagus anteriorly (this opens a window, facilitating the suturing of limbs).

Approximate limbs (two to three sutures, using the same thread as in an open procedure). These sutures are the single most difficult step in fundoplication. If they are too narrow, there is a risk of dysphagia; if they are too wide, herniation of the stomach into the mediastinum may occur. A wide bougie should therefore be inserted for calibration.

Remove the bougie for plication of the stomach posterior to the esophagus. Leave the fundus in place, checking whether it stays in position without being held.

Continued on p. 72

Fundoplication (360° Nissen)

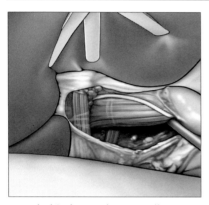

enter behind oesophagus, pull
window open

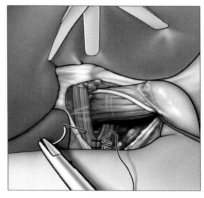

use sling, place 2-3 sutures

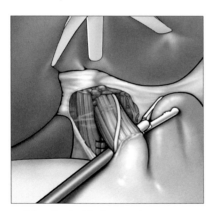

pull fundus behind oesophagus

Fundoplication (360° Nissen)

72 Apply the "shoeshine" test and push the bougie forward again. Place three sutures, loose and short. Remove the bougie and replace with a standard nasogastric tube for 24 h.

Fundoplication (360° Nissen)

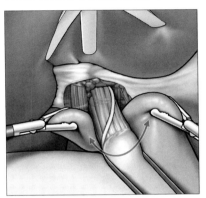 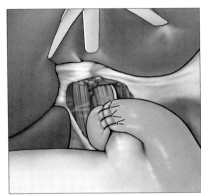

"shoe-shine test"   3 sutures

Inguineal Hernia

74 In small children (weighing 3 kg and less), reduce the bladder size by manual pressure preoperatively.

Place the monitor opposite the surgeon, on the side of the hernia. Insert the laparoscope at the umbilicus. Place two 2-mm trocars at the level of the umbilicus, lateral to the rectus muscle. Change sides for bilateral hernias. Always stand on the opposite side from the hernia. Surprisingly, contralateral sides are open in 15%-30% of patients. We close these hernias.

Continued on p. 76

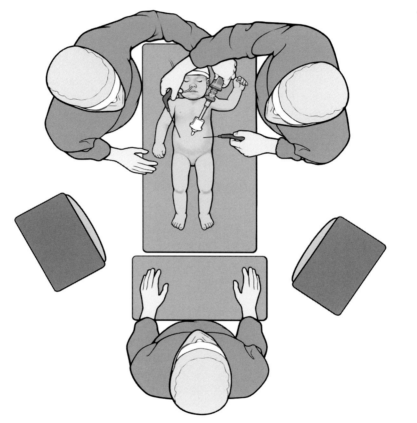

theater layout - trocar placement

Inguineal Hernia

76   Only two needle holders and a pair of scissors are required. Use a regular non-absorbable 4-0 suture with a cutting needle. Cutting needles have a better grip in the needle driver. Shorten the thread to 7 cm. Advance the needle through the abdominal wall directly above the inner inguinal ring and pull it inside with a laparoscopic needle driver.

Place the suture in an "N"-shaped fashion, and grab some underlying tissue, not only the peritoneum.

Another stitch may be required medially. Remember that hernias recur medially, next to the epigastric vessels.

Continued on p. 78

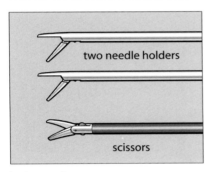

two needle holders

scissors

instruments

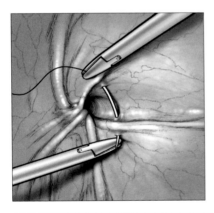 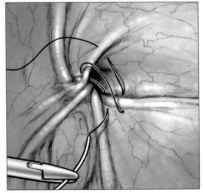

Inguineal Hernia

78   In addition, you should also include some tissue medial to the epigastric vessels and from the area between the vas and the testicular vessels.

Leave the knotted thread in place and finish the other side, if
required. Grab the two strands of each side with a needle driver,
cut the thread with a pair of scissors, and remove the sutures
together with the trocars on each side.

Direct and femoral hernias are identified during laparoscopy far
more frequently than during open surgery. They are especially frequent in recurrences after open herniotomy.

Continued on p. 80

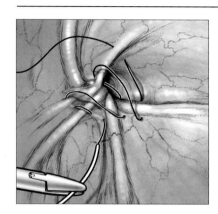 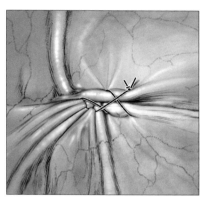

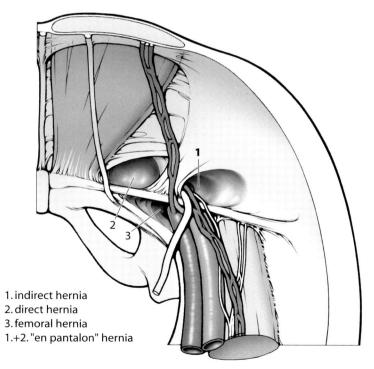

1. indirect hernia
2. direct hernia
3. femoral hernia
1.+2. "en pantalon" hernia

Inguineal Hernia

80   Direct hernias are found medial to the epigastric vessels, above the inguinal ligament. Simple closure of direct hernias (as performed in indirect hernias) carries a 50% risk of recurrence. It is advisable to open the overlying peritoneum and suture muscle and fascia tissue.

Femoral hernias are also located medially, but below the inguinal ligament. Femoral hernias are closed in an identical fashion to indirect hernias.

Combinations of direct and indirect hernias, so-called en pantalon hernias, sometimes occur. We have only seen two patients with this combination and simply sutured them.

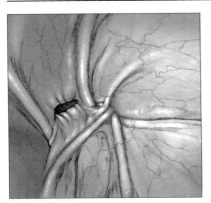

direct hernia

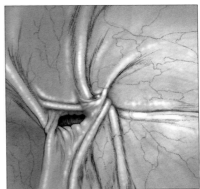

femoral hernia

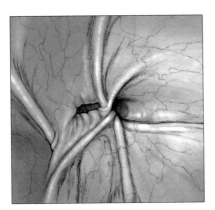

"en pantalon" hernia

Intussusception

82   Laparoscopy is suitable for those intussusceptions which are incompletely or questionably reduced radiologically.
A 5-mm laparoscope is inserted at the umbilicus. Two 2-mm trocars are advanced through the left middle abdomen and the lower mid-abdomen (the position of 2-mm trocars or their repositioning is irrelevant, since they leave virtually no scars).

Continued on p. 84

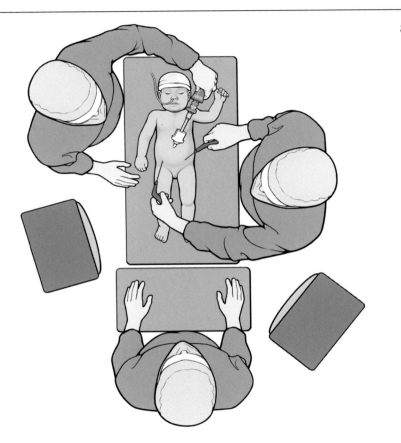

theater layout - trocar placement

Intussusception

84   You only require one set of forceps to hold the cecum and another to pull the ileum. The cecum tolerates forceps with teeth. We use forceps for bipolar coagulation on the ileum because of its blunt branches.

Some intussusceptions spontaneously reduce upon laparoscopy. Completeness is documented and the procedure terminated. Others can be reduced by pulling. If pulling and pushing with 2-mm instruments is unsuccessful, we try using 5-mm instruments. If this fails, we convert to an open approach.

Continued on p. 86

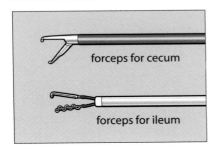

forceps for cecum

forceps for ileum

instruments

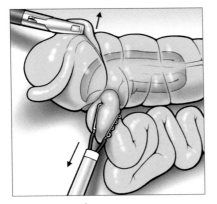

intussuscepted

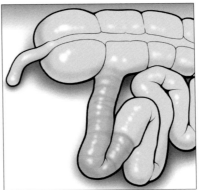

reduced

Intussusception

86   Laparoscopy is performed in patients in whom hydrostatic reduction is probably or definitively incomplete or where there is bowel "hanging" in the cecum.

With long segments of intussuscepted bowel reaching into the transverse colon or even further down, or in children with distended abdomen or peritonitis, we prefer the conventional, open approach.

Intussusception

approach

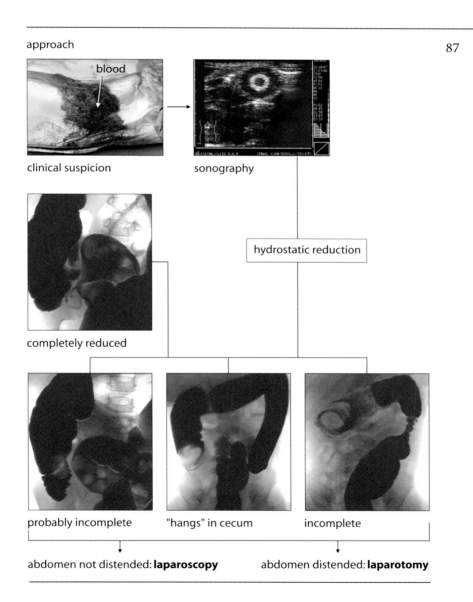

clinical suspicion

blood

sonography

hydrostatic reduction

completely reduced

probably incomplete

"hangs" in cecum

incomplete

abdomen not distended: **laparoscopy**

abdomen distended: **laparotomy**

Liver Biopsy

88   Insert the laparoscope at the umbilicus and a second 5-mm trocar
      either to the right or to the left of the umbilicus (we usually enter
      approximately 7 cm to the left of the umbilicus). No further trocars
      are needed.

Continued on p. 90

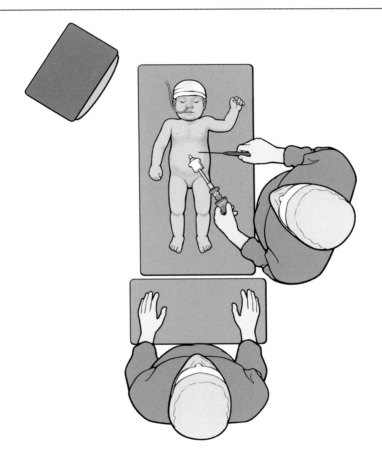

theater layout - trocar placement

Liver Biopsy

90   The instruments required are scissors, forceps with teeth to grab the excised specimen, and bipolar coagulation forceps. Check the bipolar coagulation forceps with a wet sponge prior to inserting the first trocar.

Hold the scissors with open branches against the margin of the liver.

Push the liver gently to the right.

Incise and then let go. The liver moves back to its original position.

Continued on p. 92

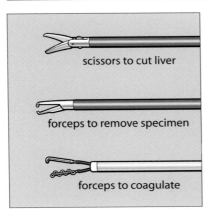

instruments

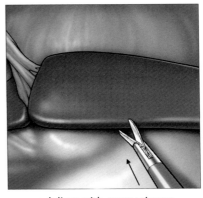

approach liver with open scissors

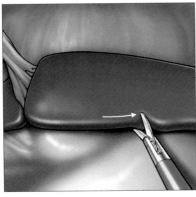

push liver laterally with open scissors

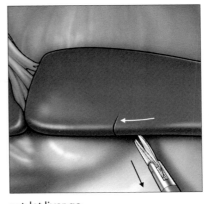

cut, let liver go

Liver Biopsy

---

92 Make the second incision shaped like an inverted "V". Do not completely excise the specimen; a small tissue bridge should be left.

Use the forceps with teeth to disrupt the last small tissue bridge and exteriorize the specimen.

Come back with the bipolar forceps and coagulate. Livers in patients with storage diseases appear to bleed less than normal livers.

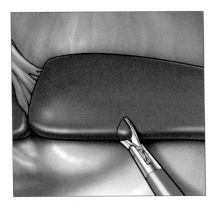

make second cut

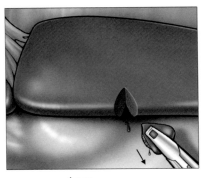

remove specimen

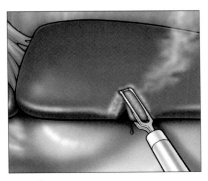

coagulate

Meckel's Diverticulum

94   If there is clinical suspicion of a Meckel's diverticulum, we abandon performing "Meckel scans" and proceed directly to laparoscopy instead.

Meckel's diverticulum might be overlooked. We therefore retrogradely check the small bowel two or three times, starting from the ileocecal area, in order not to miss a diverticulum.

Continued on p. 96

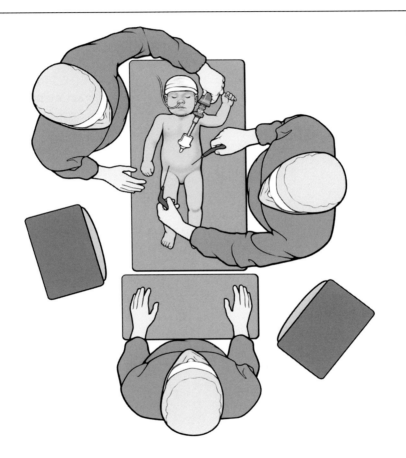

theater layout - trocar placement

Meckel's Diverticulum

96   Trocars are inserted as in appendectomy or in intussusception.
Forceps with teeth are required to hold the tip of Meckel's diverticulum, bipolar forceps are used for coagulation, and scissors are
used to transect the diverticulum.

A narrow-based Meckel's diverticulum may be ligated similarly to
an appendix, leaving an everted stump. This can be done using
5-mm instruments and endoloops alone.

Continued on p. 98

Meckel's Diverticulum

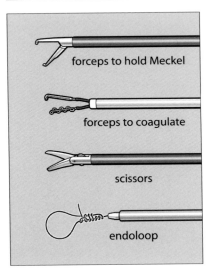

forceps to hold Meckel

forceps to coagulate

scissors

endoloop

instruments

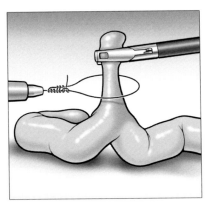

endoloop

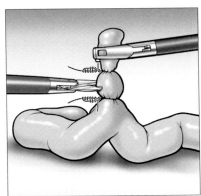

cut between endoloops

Meckel's Diverticulum

98   A broad-based Meckel's diverticulum may be removed with a stapler. Staplers require 12-mm trocars, and they leave metallic deposits in the abdomen for life.

Alternatively, the incision at the umbilicus may be spread large enough to exteriorize the Meckel's diverticulum and perform a regular "open" resection. If in doubt, we use the latter technique.

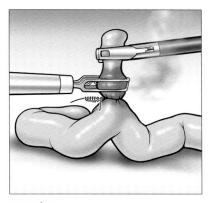

coagulate

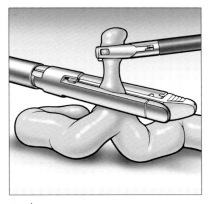

stapler

Ovary

100   Ovarian cysts in newborns usually decrease in size spontaneously with time. If a cyst of more than 4 cm in diameter remains unchanged or even appears to enlarge, we suggest laparoscopic fenestration.

The laparoscope is inserted through the umbilicus. Additional trocars are advanced into the mid-abdomen at the level of the umbilicus (or even slightly more cranially).

Continued on p. 102

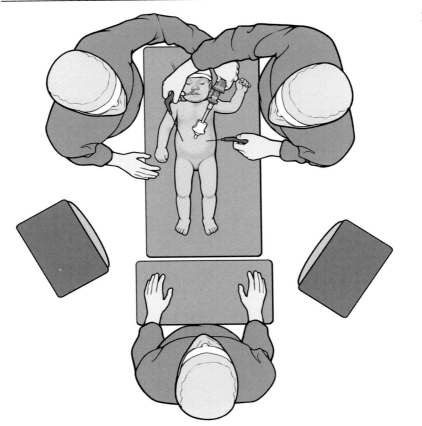

theater layout - trocar placement

Ovary

102 Forceps with teeth, blunt forceps, and a pair of scissors for incising the cyst are required. A regular long aspiration needle may also be required. These needles may damage the valve of the 2-mm trocars and create a gas leak if inserted several times.

The first view of the cyst is confusing because the laparoscope is too close for immediate orientation. The color of the cyst differs from the remaining small bowel; it is either brownish or whitish.

Brown cysts contain coagulated blood.

Continued on p. 104

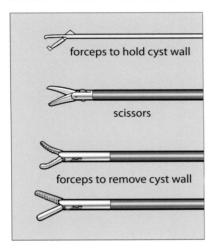

instruments

cysts in newborns

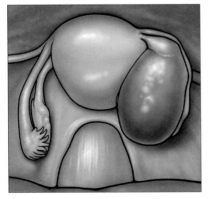

two varieties: brown...

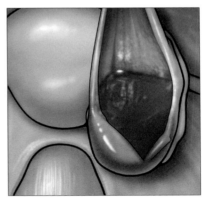

open window of the brown one

Ovary

104 White cysts contain clear or slightly yellowish liquid (hormones). The cyst is aspirated or incised. It collapses and permits orientation.

In newborns, it suffices to simply cut a window into the cyst wall. In older children, the cyst wall is incised. The two-layered wall structure becomes visible, and the inner layer can be separated from the outer layer and removed without much difficulty.

Continued on p. 106

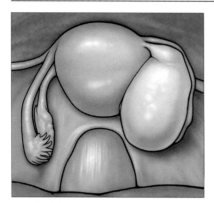 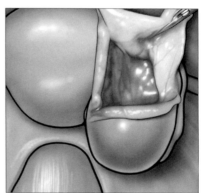

... and white   open window of the white one

cysts in older children

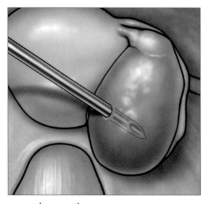 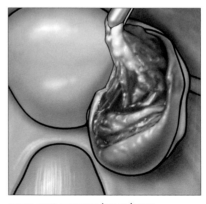

cannula empties cyst   open cyst, remove inner layer

Ovary

Torsions are readily detected. We suggest detorquing, opening a window into the cyst, and waiting. If in doubt, we return for a second laparoscopic look in approximately 3 days. Most ovaries will have recovered by then and may be left in place. We are afraid we may have removed too many ovaries in the past.

If the ovary looks histologically suspicious, we convert to an adequate incision in the lower abdomen and retrieve the specimen in an "open" procedure.

In older girls, blood in the pelvis and hemangioma-like lesions at the bladder wall or bowel wall may indicate endometriosis. The affected area needs to be excised.

torsions

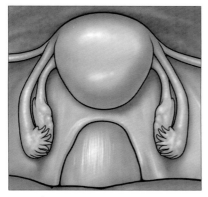

normal

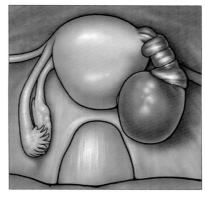

torsion

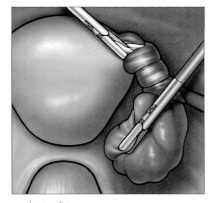

aspirate, detorque

Pyloromyotomy

108   The monitor is placed at the right side of the child's head (as in cholecystectomy). The surgeon stands on the left side, opposite the monitor.

Continued on p. 110

Pyloromyotomy

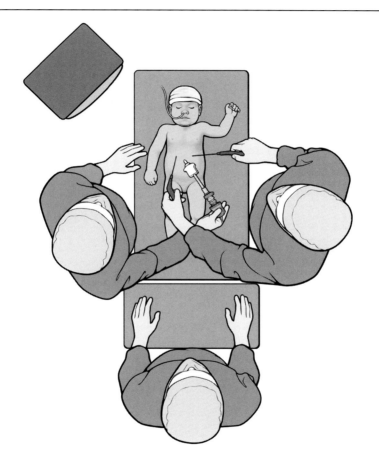

theater layout - trocar placement

Pyloromyotomy

110   A knife is required for incising the pylorus. We use a 1.7-mm blade which coagulates at the same time. The duodenum is held using 2-mm forceps with teeth. Two-millimeter instruments are too weak to spread the thickened muscle. We therefore insert a 3-mm spreader without a trocar, directly through the abdominal wall.

A 5-mm laparoscope is inserted at the umbilicus (at the infraumbilical side, as usual). The 2-mm forceps with teeth are inserted in the right upper abdomen and are used to grab the duodenum and rotate it, thereby exposing an avascular segment of the pylorus. The forceps were originally designed for use by gynecologists and have rather long teeth. The pylorus is incised with a 1.7-mm monopolar scalpel which coagulates while cutting. The knife is inserted through the left upper abdomen at the lateral margin of the rectus muscle. If the insertion is too lateral, the angle of attack will be too flat; if it is too medial, only the tip of the knife will be inserted. We have no experience of using the knives specially designed for pyloromyotomy. Some surgeons use knives designed for arthroscopy, but there is a risk of cutting too deeply. In practice, perforations occur during spreading, not during cutting.

Some laparoscopists hold the stomach through the trocar in the left upper abdomen and incise and spread the incised tissue through the right abdomen (i.e., they spread the tissue using their left hand). Right-handers prefer to perform this risky part of the operation using their right hand. There are no 2-mm spreaders on the market. The commercially available spreaders are 3 mm in diameter. We insert them directly through the abdominal wall without trocars. We prefer spreaders which have a rim at the outside of the jaws. Be careful when spreading, as the jaws tend to slip between muscle and mucosa. Most laparoscopists have a higher perforation rate in laparoscopy than with the open approach.

The postoperative feeding regimen can be resumed sooner and is more liberal than after an open approach, and hospitals usually discharge patients earlier.

Pyloromyotomy

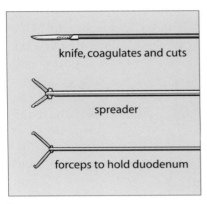

knife, coagulates and cuts

spreader

forceps to hold duodenum

instruments

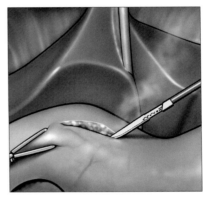

incise and coagulate

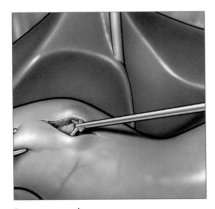

3-mm spreader

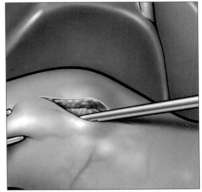

check for intact mucosa

Sigmoid Resection

Keith Georgeson

---

112 Laparoscopic Part

The complete lower body is prepped and taped. A towel at the anus controls intraoperative stool spillage. The monitor is placed near the left leg. The surgeon stands on the right, the assistant on the left side. The laparoscope (30°) is placed at the right upper abdomen. Further trocars are inserted through the umbilicus and above the cecum.

Continued on p. 114

Sigmoid Resection

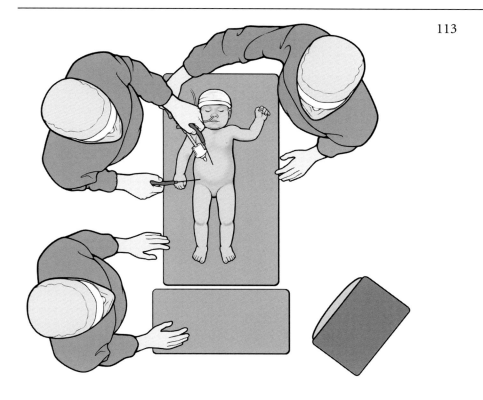

theater layout - trocar placement

Sigmoid Resection

114   Tilt the table to head down. Remove the small bowel from the pelvis. Take a biopsy with forceps and scissors. Be prepared to suture the defect.

Coagulate the sigmoid meso with a hook. Pull the hook towards you. Open a window for orientation. Stay 5 mm away from the bowel wall. Preserve the marginal artery along the bowel wall. Ligate bigger vessels with 4-0 ligatures.

At the rectum begin with the posterior wall of the rectum. Do not proceed too deeply anteriorly (1-2 cm beyond the peritoneal reflection).

Perineal Part

Pull the anus open with sutures (2-0). Suture through dentate line and arrange sutures radially outside.

Mark a circumferential line with the tip of the cautery, 0.5-1 cm above the dentate line. Incise along the line first with the cautery and then using scissors. Separate mucosa from serosa. Grab mucosa with 4-0 stay sutures, using four sutures or more. Pull the inner layer (mucosa) down. Grab some muscle with the first caudal stitches (to provide a better grip). Two millimeters higher up, move down to the mucosa proper. Moving orally, slowly separate both layers step by step, alternatively by cutting or by blunt dissection.

Apply more and more stay sutures for the mucosa as needed. Be anatomically very careful, divide each muscle fiber separately. Don't pull too hard. If a muscle fiber sticks, cut it with scissors until further pulling is possible. There is little bleeding in the plane.

Dissect approximately 7 cm of the mucosa. The transition from less perfused to normally vascularized bowel is readily seen, as is the biopsy site. When sufficiently dissected orally, grab the posterior deflection line with two Allis clamps. Cut along the line between the clamps by electrocautery.

Continued on p. 116

Sigmoid Resection

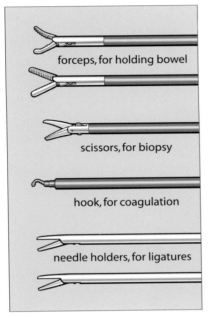

instruments

forceps, for holding bowel

scissors, for biopsy

hook, for coagulation

needle holders, for ligatures

laparoscopic part

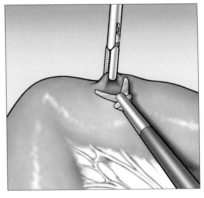

biopsy

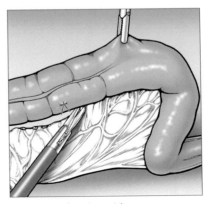

dissecting the sigmoid

Sigmoid Resection

116   Insert a finger for orientation. Complete the transection circumferentially using scissors. Incise the musculature on the back side of the tunnel in order to provide more space for the bowel to be pulled through.

Pull the bowel through. Transect the anterior part, make the anastomosis with 4-0 ligatures, then do the posterior part.

Release the stay sutures to close the anus.

Check laparoscopically for torsion or bleeding. Suturing of the peritoneum reduces the risk of a subsequent internal hernia.

Approach

Biopsy: aganglionosis

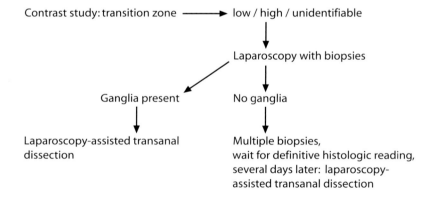

Sigmoid Resection

perineal part

dissecting the mucosa

cut

cut

Splenectomy

David van der Zee

118 Two positions are possible: right lateral or semilateral (supine position with a 30-40° tilt of the left side). The table is flexed 20-30° and elevated in a 30° anti-Trendelenburg position. The left arm is fixed in an overhead position.

The 'semilateral' position is preferred by the author. It is easier to move the table in a left or right lateral position. Also, stomach and colon will fall to the right side.

Surgeon and assistant stand on the right side of the patient, the scrubnurse on the left. One monitor is placed opposite the surgeon, the second one opposite the scrubnurse. All cables are led to the left side of the patient. A magnetic mat may be placed on the patient's thigh to prevent instruments from falling down.

Continued on p. 120

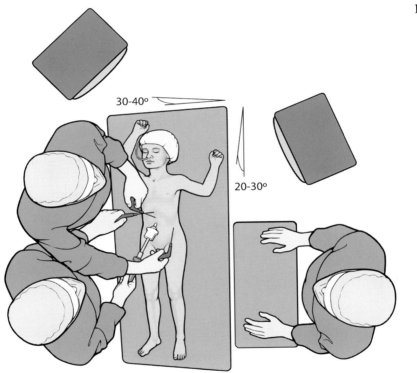

30-40°

20-30°

theater layout - trocar placement

Splenectomy

120   The first trocar is a 12 mm disposible and is placed in the subumbilical fold. This trocar is used for a 5 mm 30° optic. A 10 mm optic may optionally be used, but the advantage of a 5 mm optic is that it may be freely moved to other port sites. The 12 mm port can also be used for a 5 or 10 mm clip applier, and for the EndoGIA stapler. After removal of the trocar, a 15 mm Endobag for retrieval of the spleen can be introduced through the defect.

One trocar is placed in epigastrio for a flexible spleen retractor. The two other trocars are placed in a triangle with the first trocar, i.e. halfway between the umbilicus and xyphoid and in the anterior axillary line.

Lift the spleen either by putting the flexible spleen retractor underneath the spleen or by circumferencing the stalk of the spleen.

Retract the colon downward and dissect the splenocolic ligament by (mono- or bipolar) electrocautery or with the harmonic scalpel. By opening the lesser omental sac, the splenic vessels are displayed. Check for accessory spleens.

Continued on p. 122

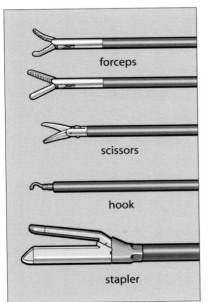

forceps

scissors

hook

stapler

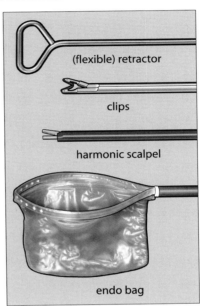

(flexible) retractor

clips

harmonic scalpel

endo bag

instruments

Splenectomy

122   The splenic vessels are dissected proximally. The vein is usually lying anterocaudal from the artery. By mobilizing the vein the artery can be reached, mobilized and transsected by ligatures, clips or by using the harmonic scalpel or EndoGIA. Thereafter, the vein is transsected. Sometimes the tail of the pancreas may lie high up in the hilum of the spleen requiring a more extensive dissection. In this case, transsection of the vessels at a more distal position, especially when using the harmonic scalpel, may be easier.

Now dissect the gastroepiploic and short gastric vessels. Proceed with care. Don't rush. Transsect each vessel separately after sufficient mobilization. Transsect the remaining peritoneal attachments.

The optic is now moved to the port halfway between umbilicus and xyphoid and the 12 mm trocar in the umbilicus is removed. A 15 mm Endobag is introduced through the opening. By laying the ring of the Endobag on the medial side of the spleen, after opening the ring, the spleen can usually be scooped into the bag by a lateral movement. In this way the omentum or small intestines usually do not interfere. In case of a large spleen this procedure may be more tedious. In this case it may be advantageous to introduce the caudal pole of the spleen into the Endobag and then release the bag of the ring and further manually pull the sac around the spleen towards the top.

After the spleen has been caught in the sac the suture around the sac can be pulled. The sac is moved to the umbilicus. If a morcellator is used the opening of the sac is pulled out through the umbilicus. If the finger-fracture method is used, the fascia should be incised up to 4-5 cm to allow two digits to be introduced into the abdomen, before pulling the bag out of the umbilicus. The finger-fracture method is used by the author because of its simplicity and speed. Care should be taken to keep the opening of the sac well above the wound to avoid spillage.

In case of cholelithiasis the table may be turned over to the left to give adequate exposure of the right subcostal area. One additional trocar in the right subcostal region is sufficient for either cholecystotomy with stone removal or for cholecystectomy.

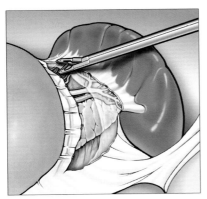

transsection of vessels with clips

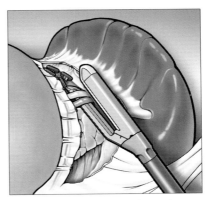

transsection of vessels with stapler

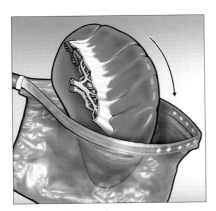

scooping of the spleen

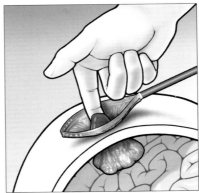

finger fracture

Varicocele

124   Most varicoceles are left-sided. The monitor is therefore placed
next to the patient's left thigh. The surgeon stands to the right of
the patient. A 5-mm laparoscope is placed through the umbilicus,
and a 2-mm trocar is inserted at the level of the umbilicus at the
lateral margin of the rectus muscle. This is a relatively avascular
area. Going through the rectus muscle carries the risk of bleeding.
A second 2-mm trocar is inserted above the bladder in an area likely to be covered later by pubic hair.

Continued on p. 126

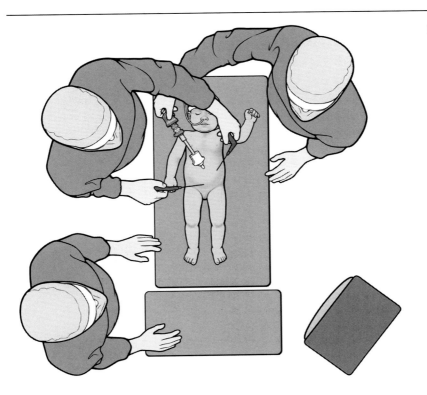

theater layout - trocar placement

Varicocele

126 The instruments required are forceps to lift the peritoneum above the vessels and to dissect the vessels, scissors to incise the peritoneum and transect the vessels, and two 2-mm needle holders to ligate the vessels.

The ectatic veins are easily seen, even with an intraabdominal pressure of 12 mmHg. Comparison with the contralateral side confirms the diagnosis. In varicoceles, there is often adhesion of the sigmoid colon to the peritoneum covering the varicocele. Transecting or pulling off the adhesion results in small areas of bleeding, rendering the picture unclear.

We incise the peritoneum in the shape of a "T". The artery is often buried below a bundle of veins. When touched with forceps, the artery tends to constrict and is subsequently impossible to distinguish from the veins. Be careful to avoid even the smallest amount of bleeding when dissecting the veins, as bleeding makes it impossible to identify the artery. We try to preserve the artery.

If bleeding occurs, the only option may be to ligate the whole bundle, both the artery and the veins. In probably 30% of cases, it is impossible to identify the artery despite the use of Doppler sonography and pharmacologic agents. We are uncertain which technique is best. If the artery is preserved, there are fewer hydroceles, but recurrences may be more frequent. If the artery is transected, there might be fewer recurrences, but more hydroceles.

We ligate the vessels with nonabsorbable ligatures. Clips (used by many laparoscopists because they are quick to apply) require at least 5-mm trocars. We transected the vessels after ligating in some patients, while in others we did not.

We coagulated the vessels after ligature in several patients. In two patients, a zone of hypoesthesia or hyperesthesia was noted at the thigh postoperatively ("meralgia"), but it subsided after a few weeks. An underlying nerve had obviously been damaged during coagulation. If you keep one hand on the patient's thigh while coagulating vessels, you will notice any nerve damage immediately because the thigh moves.

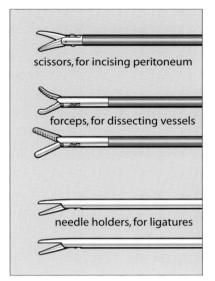

instruments

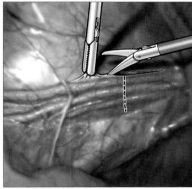

incision of peritoneum

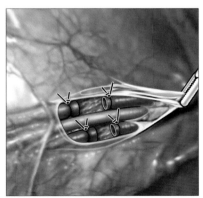

separated, ligated veins,
artery preserved

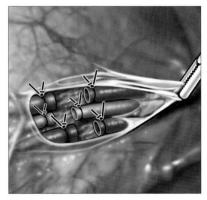

artery not preserved, 2-mm ligatures

Thoracoscopy

128 Lung biopsies and mediastinal masses were our most frequent thoracoscopic procedures in children. For unilateral ventilation see the chapter on anesthesia.

Position and tilt the patient in such a way that gravity pulls the collapsed lung away from your target area. Place the trocar for the 5-mm scope like a chest tube (skin incision, spreading with scissors, blunt advancement). Wait a minute for the lung to collapse. Usually, we insufflate CO_2 at 0.3 L/min up to 7 mmHg in order to speed up the collapsing. Too aggressive insufflating may result in bradycardia.

Continued on p. 130

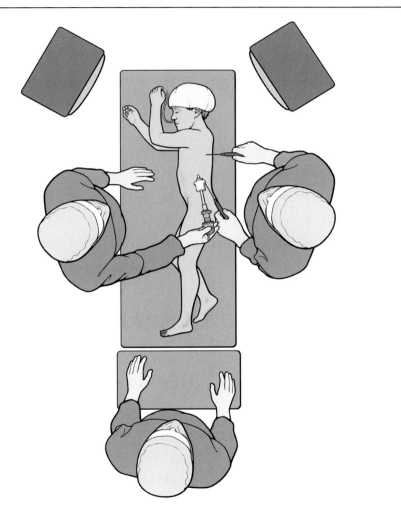

theater layout - trocar placement, lateral positioning for thoracoscopy

Thoracoscopy

130 Lung Biopsy

Biopsies at the lung periphery are easy. Biopsies of central parts of the lung are better performed in the "open" technique.

Insert the scope near the intended biopsy. Insert two trocars at least 5 cm apart from the scope.

a) Using an Endoloop: Use 5-mm trocars. Insert an Endoloop through the right trocar. With the left hand, pull the lung tissue through the loop and close the loop.

b) Using staplers: Use the required trocar for the stapler on the right side (10 or 12 mm). Grab the lung as in (a).

The suture line looks better with staplers. However, metallic foreign bodies are left behind.

With Endoloops the tissue looks tied up.

When finished, the lung is insufflated until it almost prolapses into the trocar. No drainage is required. The fascia and the skin are sutured.

Continued on p. 132

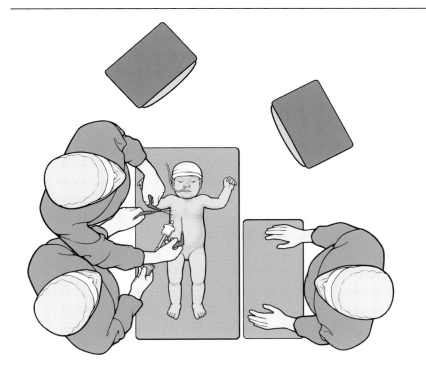

theater layout - trocar placement, supine positioning for thoracoscopy

Thoracoscopy

---

132 Mediastinal Masses

Patients are in supine position. Mind the phrenic nerve, which often crosses the tumor. Practically all the teratoma rupture at some point, and are eventually removed within a bag through the lowest and most posterior incision. Dissecting and transsecting are very much like "open" surgery.

Pneumothorax

Open the bullae with scissors. This exposes raw lung surface with fistulae. Cover the surface and the fistulae with fibrin glue or fleece like Tachocomb.

Continued on p. 134

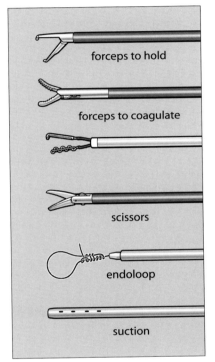

forceps to hold

forceps to coagulate

scissors

endoloop

suction

instruments

biopsy

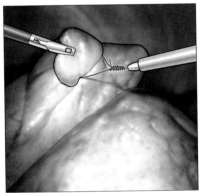

134 Sympathectomy

The patient is in supine position with both arms extended at 90°. Insert a 5-mm scope below the axilla and one or two additional 2-mm trocars laterally. One trocar should suffice, the second may be needed to keep the lung away. Wait a minute for the lung to collapse. For hyperhidrosis of the hands only, coagulate ganglia 2 and 3. For the axilla, coagulate ganglion 4. The ganglia are easily identified as a white, cord-like structure crossing the paravertebral ribs. Cave: destroying ganglion 1 results in Horner's syndrome.

We have coagulated the ganglia with a laser fiber. This requires only a scope and a 12-gauge needle; the fiber is small enough to be passed though a regular 12-gauge hypodermic needle. However, the needle tip swings too much. Precise aiming is difficult. Furthermore, the laser makes smog inside the thorax, leading to impaired vision. We also had bleeding from an intercostal vessel that was injured by the laser.

In other patients, we have transsected the ganglia with 2-mm scissors. In further patients, we have coagulated the ganglia with a 2-mm forceps. Coagulating is quickest. The series is too small to conclude which technique is best.

Remember that 30-40% of patients will have "compensatory sweating" at the back or the abdomen.

pneumothorax

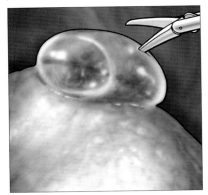

open bulla

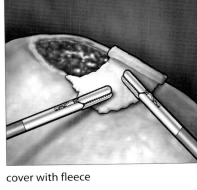

cover with fleece

mediastinal tumor

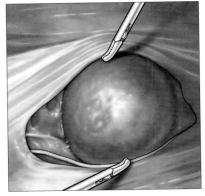

opened pleura

sympathectomy

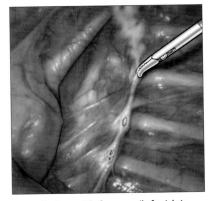

coagulation with forceps (left side)

Trouble Shooting: Who, What, When?

136   **The Day Before Laparoscopy**

Surgeon

- Be prepared
- Take courses, read journals and practice
- Be able to cope with complications: (trocar injuries to great vessels, Veres needle lesions of organs)

Patient

- Obtain informed consent
- Prepare for a possible transfusion (cross-match)
- Take previous surgery into account (adhesions)
- Consider other reasons for a dilated bowel (stenosis, dysganglionosis)
- Consider an enema (to collapse a distended large bowel, although we believe this is unnecessary)
- Ask the patient to urinate immediately prior to going to the operating room

Nurse

The nurse should:
- Be familiar with the technique
- Be ready to cope with a quick conversion to an open procedure
- Know who will change the CO_2 bottle during the procedure
- Check that all the instruments are ready

Anesthesiologist

The anesthesiologist should be prepared for:
- A lengthy procedure
- The risk of bleeding
- The risk of gas embolus

Trouble Shooting: Who, What, When?

- Is the cautery functioning? (important in critical situations)
- Is the imaging working? (colors)
- Do all the cables fit?

Patient on the Table

Surgeon

- Check whether all the instruments are available.
- Ask the nurse to check the instruments while you are looking on.
- Ask him or her to close all the valves on the trocars (they come from the factory with open valves, and open valves will immediately desufflate CO_2 and increase the risk of organ puncture).
- Check whether there are enough reduction valves (for 10- to 5-mm trocars) and whether they are from the same manufacturer.
- Check the type of laparoscope (0°/30°/45°?) and its diameter (5 or 10 mm?). You want 5 mm/0° or 30°.
- Check whether there are enough CO_2 bottles in reserve.
- Establish where the monitors will be placed (in a straight line, opposite the surgeon).
- Find out who will help you if something goes wrong (write down phone numbers).

Assistant

- Work quietly and slowly.
- If bleeding occurs, pull the laparoscope back slightly, but do not change the view.
  Point ZERO upward (avoid rotating the laparoscope).

Trouble Shooting: Who, What, When?

Anesthesiologist

- Check that the patient is relaxed.
- The ether screen should be as low as possible (space for manipulating the laparoscope in the pelvis).
- You should know where the controls are for adjusting the table.

Patient

- Consider use of an urinary catheter (we believe this is unnecessary).
- Consider use of a nasogastric tube (probably better).
- Put a neutral electrode in place (for emergency/conversion).
- Check positioning (the patient should be fixed to the table in such a way that intraoperative rotation and tilting is possible).
- There should be no padding (it brings the vertebral column and the large vessels dangerously close to the trocars).
- If an adhesiolysis is scheduled, lift the patient up (so that instruments can be lowered enough to reach the anterior wall from the inside, operation "at the ceiling").

Prepping

- Prepare for a possible conversion to an open procedure.
- The surgeon should not become entangled in light and CO_2 cables (intraoperative change of sides should be possible).

Trouble Shooting: Who, What, When?

Difficulties in Positioning the Veres Needle

- Check the needle prior to insertion to ensure it is working properly (may not slide well and not fully open at the tip, thus blocking gas flow).
- Lift the abdominal wall during insertion.
- Check you really are deep enough (noticeable/audible snap when penetrating fascia).
- If the needle is not erect, the lateral opening may be obstructed by peritoneum (indicated by high pressure, no flow).
- If uncertain, aspirate, withdraw, and insert the needle again.

Problems with CO_2 Flow

Status	Most likely cause	Action
High pressure (>15 mmHg), no flow	Wrong positioning of needle (not intraperitoneal)	Withdraw
	Any valve closed (mostly at the trocar)	Open valve
	CO_2 bottle closed	Open bottle
	Tubes disconnected	Connect
Low pressure (>5 mmHg), high flow	Leak	
	Trocar slipped out	Reinsert, fixate
	Instrument and trocar do not fit	Remove instrument
	Leak around the (usually tilted) trocar	Purse string

140 *Cautery*

Prior to inserting the Veres needle or trocar, check coagulation by coagulating a wet sponge (this only works with bipolar coagulation; you cannot check monopolar cautery). Remember that the cautery is the most frequent cause of problems. This piece of equipment is the one that fails most often, and it is the most difficult one to handle.

Veres Needle

- Reusable (check free flow with saline) or disposable needles (disposable ones are more expensive)?
- Does the protective mechanism slide?
- Incise the skin first, nick the fascia.
- Lift the abdominal wall. (Is the patient relaxed?)
- Insert the needle obliquely.
- Make sure it snaps in place.
- Aspirate and perform the "hanging drop" test.
- Start with a low flow.
- If there is no flow or if you are uncertain, withdraw the needle.
- Consider other positions.

Fogging of the Laparoscope

There are several options if fogging of the laparoscope occurs:
- Wait until system warms up and fogging disappears spontaneously.
- Place the laparoscope in hot water for a few minutes (best option).
- Place the laparoscope into an autoclave shortly before surgery.
- Buy a special heater.

Trouble Shooting: Who, What, When?

- Briefly touch the mesentery or peritoneum inside the abdomen
  (this may work for a few seconds, but may also smear the optic
  and make things worse).
- Use a household detergent (this works, but it is not readily available in sterile form).
- Use a commercially available anti-fogging substance or alcohol
  for skin desinfection (works well).

No Picture or Bad Picture

The best protection is to check personally prior to surgery. Otherwise, ensure that a technician is available. Pictures are often bad when you desperately need good ones. "White balance" is only required when changing laparoscope sizes or manufacturers.

Full Bladder

A full bladder can be ignored, because it does not impair most procedures. Exceptions are diagnostic procedures at the inner genitalia. If necessary, insert a needle through the anterior wall under view and evacuate the bladder or (in small children) express the bladder manually.

Omentum Hanging Up at the Anterior Abdominal Wall

If the omentum is hanging up at the anterior abdominal wall, this indicates that the Veres needle was too deep and insufflated beneath the omentum. This can be ignored, because it will gradually fall down. Alternatively, it can be pulled down using an instrument through the second trocar.

Trouble Shooting: Who, What, When?

Abdominal Wall Thickened by Gas Emphysema

If the abdominal wall is thickened by gas emphysema, this indicates that the Veres needle was not deep enough and insufflated outside the peritoneum. The surgeon can ignore this and carry on with the operation. The emphysema will disappear within 10 min.

Bowel Distended, No View

A distended bowel blocking the view is characteristic in small children and is most prominent in the transverse colon in fundoplication. The surgeon can either carry on with surgery or wait until it has decreased.

Trocars

Reusable trocars are more cost-effective, but become blunt and quickly become out of date. Disposable ones are costly, but they are always sharp, always work, and are easily replaced by better ones. As a compromise, the first (i.e., blind) trocar can be disposable, and the second/third ones reusable.

Oblique insertion is less risky. You should apply a protective finger. If the trocar is difficult to insert or appears to be stuck, check whether the snap mechanism has already moved (be aware of the danger of "rushing in" with the rearmed trocar).

Vessels likely to be damaged are the aorta/cava and the iliac. If vessel injury occurs:

- Leave the trocars in place.
- Maintain insufflation.
- Convert to an open procedure.

When the laparoscope has been inserted, first check for trocar or Veres injury.

If the optic fogs, rub it against fat or against the abdominal wall.

Trouble Shooting: Who, What, When?

If there is blood in the trocar, rinse it with saline though the valve
for insufflation.

Second and third trocars:
- Perform diaphanoscopy of the abdominal wall to avoid vessel perforation (epigastrics).
- Do not cross the umbilical ligaments (you will become entangled).
- Insert the trocar under view.
- Counteract, if necessary.

If bleeding occurs from the trocar site, replace by a bigger trocar with a balloon, block the balloon, and pull it up.

If bleeding occurs upon withdrawal of the trocar (epigastrics), use a blocking urinary catheter/suturing.

Veres needle injury is rare and difficult to identify. It affects the bowel, liver, and bladder and can be sutured laparoscopically.

In contrast, trocar injury is the single most dangerous step during laparoscopy. It affects the aorta, iliac vessels, and the inferior vena cava. It is easier to notice: large vessel injury results in the picture becoming all red, but the exact site of lesion is not visible and there is no spurting. The posterior peritoneum comes forward, and the abdominal space diminishes despite increased pressure. It requires conversion to an open procedure.

You should briefly try to grab the vessel with the forceps, but if this is unsuccessful, you should remove instruments but leave the trocars in place and leave the pressure unchanged or even increase pressure. Begin laparotomy with the trocars in situ and the pressure increased. Be aware that as soon as the peritoneum is opened, CO_2 will escape, the intraabdominal pressure will decrease, and bleeding will increase significantly.

When clamping and suturing vessels, remember that most penetrations also affect the posterior wall. The lumbar arteries should be preserved (danger of paraplegia).

144 *Bleeding During Preparation*

This is usually minor. The camera should not be moved (only slightly withdrawn). Be prepared for bleeding: always keep forceps in the vicinity. Coagulate first and suction later (suction removes CO_2, which leads to a poor view and distorts the anatomy; it appears "all red" and the vessel withdraws).

Technical Tips on Preventing Problems

- When changing instruments, hold the trocar fixed (the next instrument will arrive at the same position).
- Keep the tip of instruments in the center of the screen.
- Fixate trocars (using suture or tape) in babies, as they can easily fall out.
- Stay "in line" (surgeon - organ - monitor), and do not operate "around the corner".
- If you lose the needle during suturing, it is often stuck in the trocar.
- Identify where the needle tip is pointing at (a very close view will show).
- If gas is lost, remove the instruments and wait until the abdomen fills up again.
- Insert trocars away from the operative field.

Postoperative Problems

Shoulder pain may occur for 36 h (the cause is unclear, but it disappears).

Sometimes patients have an elevated temperature up to 38.5°C for 36 h (the cause is unclear, but it disappears).

"Postlaparoscopy syndrome" may also occur (the cause is unclear; it looks like peritonitis 3-4 days postoperatively, but disappears with or without antibiotics within a further 2 days).

Index

145

Index

Index